BODY
BASICS
for bones

Beat osteoporosis,
build better bones!

Here's what people are saying about
BODY BASICS *for bones*

"BODY BASICS *for bones* is an easy-to-read, informative guide that gives prevention the place it deserves. Not only does it emphasize good nutrition and other lifestyle habits, it gives practical guidelines on how to put them into practice."

TEENA VAN'T FOORT RD, M.H.Sc.
PUBLIC HEALTH NUTRITIONIST

". . . an invaluable resource for all osteoporosis treatment centers to offer their patients. . . an excellent starting point for conditioning body and bone . . . contains concise information . . . extremely helpful instructional section . . ."

Dr. ANTHONY HODSMAN M.D., FRCP
DIRECTOR, LONDON REGIONAL OSTEOPOROSIS PROGRAM

". . . finally, models that are real people . . . real ages and shapes . . . **BODY BASICS *for bones*** deals with key issues such as managing pain and what to do if you suffer a fracture . . . I look forward to starting the exercises."

LAUREL CROSS
TOWN OF THE BLUE MOUNTAINS

"I am so pleased that at last a truly helpful book will be available to individuals who have, or who are concerned about, osteoporosis. This book allows the public to read solid information at home and then take the personal action necessary to combat this debilitating disease."

GAIL LEMIEUX
WOMAN WITH OSTEOPOROSIS
DIRECTOR, OSTEOPOROSIS SOCIETY OF CANADA 1997-2000

"I will be recommending this book in both my clinical practice as well as my continuing education workshops for physiotherapists, fitness leaders and nurses."

KATHY BOUCHARD B.Sc.(KIN); B.Sc.(PT)
OSTEOPOROSIS SPECIALIST

"A great guide for osteoporosis prevention . . . photographs with clear instructions make the exercises easy to follow."

DR. ALEXANDRA PAPAIOANNOU M.D., FRCPC
ASSOCIATE PROFESSOR, DEPARTMENT OF MEDICINE
McMASTER UNIVERSITY

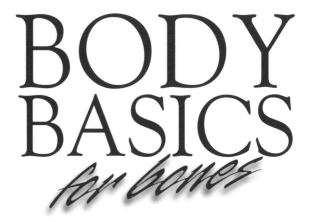

BODY BASICS for bones

Beat osteoporosis,
build better bones!

Karen Webb B.P.T., MCPA
Dr. Darien Lazowski Ph.D., B.Sc. P.T.

Birchcliff Publishing Inc.
Thornbury, Ontario, Canada

Body Basics *for life* is a trademark of Birchcliff Publishing Inc.

Canadian Cataloguing in Publication Data.

Webb, Karen, 1953 -
Body basics *for bones*: beat osteoporosis, build better bones!

Includes bibliographical references and index.
ISBN 0-9682571-3-5

1.Osteoporosis-Prevention. I. Lazowski, Darien-Alexis, 1957- II. Title

RC931.O73W42 2000   616.7'16   C00-900430-0

Production Art by Caroline Sweet
Photography by Mary Lynn Fluter-Shackel and Michael McClintock
Editing by Layne Verbeek
Cover and Author (K. Webb) Photo by Elisabeth Feryn
Author (D. Lazowski) Photo by Mary Lynn Fluter-Shackel
Printed in Canada by The Beacon Herald Fine Printing Division, Stratford, Ontario

All inquiries should be addressed to:
Birchcliff Publishing Inc.
Box 639
Thornbury, Ontario
N0H 2P0
(519) 599-2053
Web site www: bodybasicsforlife.com

Quantity discounts are available on bulk purchases of this book. For information contact Birchcliff Publishing Inc. at the above address or call us at (519) 599-2053 or toll-free at 1-888-472-9121. A mail-order form is located in the back of the book.

Body Basics *for bones*: Beat osteoporosis, build better bones! is not intended as medical advice. This book's intention is solely educational and informational while lending itself to prevention and self-help. The reader should regularly consult a physician in matters relating to his or her health and individual needs. Clearance from your physician is recommended prior to beginning an exercise program. The authors and the publisher expressly disclaim any liability, loss, or risk, personal or otherwise, which is incurred as a consequence, directly or indirectly, of the use and application of any of the contents of this book.

Reprint 2002

This book is dedicated to Sam, Kirstie
and their grandmother, Winifred.
It is never too early nor too late
to build better bones.

ACKNOWLEDGEMENTS

Production Art by Caroline Sweet
Photography by Mary Lynn Fluter-Shackel and
Michael McClintock
Editing by Layne Verbeek
Cover and Author (K. Webb) Photo by Elisabeth
Feryn
Author (D. Lazowski) Photo by Mary Lynn
Fluter-Shackel

Tena Van't Foort, M.H.Sc., RD is a Public Health
Nutritionist at The Bruce-Grey-Owen Sound
Health Unit. Tena has been an excellent resource
throughout the research component of this project.
Tena has provided us with nutritional information
in a timely fashion. She has also directed us to the
most current resources available in North America.

Barbara Beatty, B.Sc.P.T., an expert in the field of
osteoporosis rehabilitation, has been a great inspira-
tion and source of information for many years. Our
long and lively discussions about osteoporosis are
always enjoyable.

Kathy Shipp P.T., M.H.S., is a Physical Therapist in
the United States. Her clinical expertise in the field
of osteoporosis has been of great assistance in the
final stages and completion of this project.

And our sincere thanks go out to all the models
appearing in this book. A picture is worth a thou-
sand words! Thank You: Antonia Benjaminsen, Mike
Chandler, Terry Daniel, John Deyoung, Catherine
Diavolitsis, Maria Dolezal, Mercy Doxtator, Sarah
Fluter, Grace Hendrickson, Zachary Herlick, Doris
Hines, Anne Mullen, Linda Pigeon, Shirley
Redgwell, Audrey Smith, Anne Swinkels, Shelley
Swinkels-Herlick, Rosemary Tanner, Laila Viani,
Pamela Wardle, Kirstie Webb, Samantha Webb
Lijuan Yao, Don Young, Ellen Young, Dianne Yundt
and Wayne Yundt.

Darien would like to thank her husband, Laurence,
for his patience, wisdom, skepticism and scientific
expertise; her son, Declan, for sharing the computer
and letting mummy do her work sometimes; and all
the women with osteoporosis who have taught her
so much over the years.

CONTENTS

8 Stand Up & Bone Up

10 What is Osteoporosis & Who Gets It?

13 It's Never Too Early

15 Why We Lose Bone Mass

18 Food For Your Bones

25 Bending & Muscle Imbalances

28 Plumbline Postures

30 Sit Safely & Protect Your Spine

33 Safe & Healthy Driving

36 Everyday Life Activities

40 Medicine for Your Bones

46 Let's Walk for the Health of It

49 Let's Try Running

51 Postural Retraining: Easy Steps to Straighten Up

52 Static & Dynamic Postural Correction

54 Abdominal Strengthening

58 Back Straightening & Strengthening

61 Shoulder Straightening & Strengthening

64 Keeping Your Balance

68 Sports & Recreation

69 What to Do if You Have a Fracture

73 Pain Management

75 In Summary

76 Bibliography & Helpful Resources

78 Healthy Products

80 Mail Order

STAND UP & BONE UP

Osteoporosis is much like high blood pressure in that it develops silently. Sometimes referred to as the *silent thief*, it steals your bone mass without warning and a fracture is often the first sign of its presence. And, contrary to belief, osteoporosis is not just a disease of the elderly. Furthermore, it is never too early, nor too late, to protect you and your family from developing osteoporosis.

Osteoporosis is a rapidly growing problem that now affects millions of North Americans and most of us probably know a friend, colleague or family member who has osteoporosis. The increased frequency of osteoporosis is in part due to changing lifestyles, poorer eating habits and nutrition, decreased physical activity and a greater reliance on medications. The great number of people now heading into their fifties (boomers) is also a significant factor.

It is never too early nor too late to protect you and your family from developing osteoporosis.

Most of us have little concern about the health of our bones when we are young. We wait until we are older, slower and beginning to develop significant health problems before we take positive steps to change our diets and physical habits. Yet when it comes to our bones, our diet and levels of activity are critical - *right from the start*. The bone strength you build in childhood through young adulthood can help you have healthier bones well into your mid and later years. And even if you didn't take steps to build healthier bones when you were younger, it is never too late to start, as changes you make to your diet and activity level at any time will always help your bones.

BODY BASICS *for bones* provides you with up-to-date information and evidence-based practices to take good care of your bones. By taking the right steps *now*, you avoid becoming an older person who walks stooped forward with rounded shoulders, or someone who has to live with constant fears of chronic pain or risk of fractures. By taking control

STAND UP
& BONE UP

and making informed decisions that lead to positive changes, you will begin to build better bones and enjoy the quality of life you deserve - now and in the future.

So start now to learn the facts, make healthy choices and build better bones!

Karen Webb and Dr. Darien Lazowski

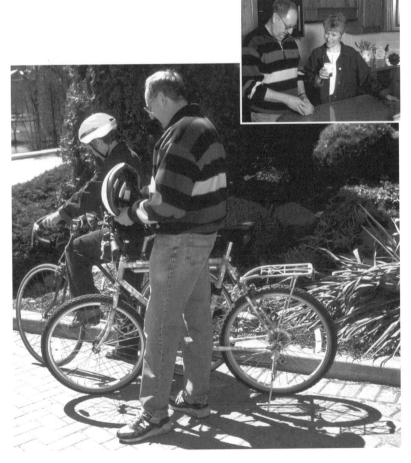

WHAT IS OSTEOPOROSIS & WHO GETS IT?

Osteoporosis means "porous bones." It mainly affects women and men over 50, with post-menopausal women being at the greatest risk. Bones become thin and weak with age, and can therefore break or fracture easily. The bones most likely to fracture are the bones in the spine, wrists, ribs and/or hips. Spinal fractures result in a progressive loss in height.

Most people don't know when they are developing osteoporosis and it often takes a fracture before the person becomes aware of its presence. Osteoporosis may surface as a sudden, severe pain in the spine of an elderly person who lifts a heavy bag of groceries out of their car or in a 35 year-old who fractures a rib after a bout of bad coughing. And, contrary to common belief, osteoporosis is neither a disease unique to the elderly nor to women only.

Nonetheless, some of us are more likely to get osteoporosis than others, as there are many genetic and other related factors that put certain people at risk. And although we cannot choose our parents, we do need to know about these risk factors. There are also certain medical conditions and medications that can increase your risk of osteoporosis and these should be discussed with your doctor and planned for appropriately. Finally, there are also a number of lifestyle and nutritional risk factors - but fortunately, these are factors over which we all have control. It is important to note that people with no risk factors may still develop osteoporosis.

You and your family's risk for osteoporosis increases with low-calcium diets, smoking, alcohol abuse and sedentary lifestyles.

WHAT IS OSTEOPOROSIS & WHO GETS IT?

RISK FACTORS FOR OSTEOPOROSIS & OSTEOPOROSIS FRACTURES

The following risk factors are noted by the Osteoporosis Society of Canada and the National Osteoporosis Foundation in the United States.

- Female sex

- Age 50 or older

- Past menopause

- Prolonged hormonal imbalances **

- Ovaries removed or menopause before age 45 **

- Not enough calcium or vitamin D in diet **

- Family history of osteoporosis **

- Personal history of fracture as an adult (with minimal trauma) **

- Smoker

- Not enough physical activity

- White or Asian ancestry

- Thin, small boned

- Caffeine (consistently more than three cups a day of coffee, tea or cola)

- Alcoholism (consistently more than two drinks a day)

- Excessive use of certain medications (cortisone and prednisone, anti-convulsants, thyroid hormone, aluminum containing antacids) **

RISK FACTORS FOR OSTEOPOROSIS & OSTEOPOROSIS FRACTURES (cont'd)

- Primary hyperparathyroidism **

- Poor health/frailty **

- Low body weight (less than 127 lb/57.8 kg) **

**STRONGER PREDICTORS

There are secondary causes of osteoporosis which include a broad range of diseases and therapeutic drugs. For more information about these causes talk to your attending physician or contact one of the organizations listed under " Helpful Resources" on page 77.

A well balanced diet rich in calcium and regular exercise are the corner-stones of building strong bones.

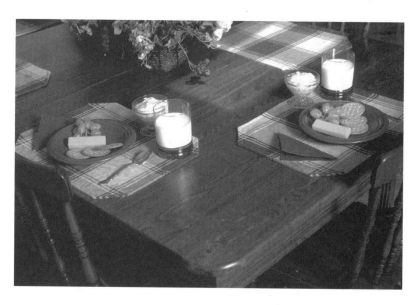

IT'S NEVER TOO EARLY

Most of our bone mass growth is likely reached during our teens and peaks when we are 30. As parents or grandparents, we need to ensure that our young people are given accurate information about maintaining the health of their bones right from the start. A well balanced diet rich in calcium and regular exercise are the cornerstones of building strong bones, for what happens during these critical early years has a tremendous impact on the health of young peoples' bones in later life.

Unfortunately, the majority of North American children do not meet their daily calcium requirements. Furthermore, children today are far less active than before as they sit for long hours in front of the television, video games and computers. Smoking can also alter their hormone levels and contribute to further bone loss. And, at the other extreme, excessive exercise, combined with inadequate nutrition, can also lead to irregular hormonal changes and loss of bone mass. So, like most things in life, we all (young and old) need to exercise and eat in moderation.

Look for calcium-fortified orange juice at your grocery store.

An additional problem is that it is often difficult to get children to take in enough calcium through their diets. Most frequently, we see teenage girls avoiding dairy products due to their fat content - even though these are the most calcium-rich foods available. So if you have any doubt your children are not getting adequate daily intakes of calcium through their diets, you should consider introducing calcium supplements. And while liquid calcium is easily available and can be added to soups or beverages, it is recommended that you talk to a registered dietitian or family doctor before taking this step.

This book includes a list of common sources of calcium with serving sizes and fat content for each source. Not everyone wants to consume a lot of dairy products, but it is important to recognize that milk is one of the best sources for calcium. One cup of milk, whether it is whole or skim, contains about the same amount of calcium (310 milligrams (mg)). Fat content varies, however, ranging from traces in skim milk to 3 grams (g) in 1%, 5 g in 2% and 9 g in whole milk (3%). Compare that to one fast food breakfast sandwich with egg and sausage that only has 155 mg of calcium but 39 grams of fat. You would have to drink 13 cups of 1% milk to get the same amount of dietary fat as the egg and sausage sandwich!

So, share your knowledge with your children and help them make good choices. For not only are healthy habits, including eating well and regular exercise, easier to develop early in life, these habits are much more likely to last.

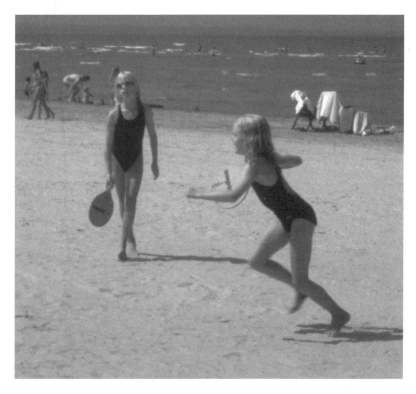

WHY WE LOSE BONE MASS

NATURAL CHANGES

Our bodies lose bone mass gradually throughout life. While the body has a natural bone maintenance process called bone remodeling (or bone turnover), where new bone is formed and old bone is taken away, this process occurs mostly during infancy and childhood and markedly slows with age. The bone strength we build in childhood and early adulthood also helps us maintain healthier bones later in life, for by the time we reach 30 years old, our bones are at their peak bone mass, which means they are as strong as they will ever be. A number of factors can influence peak bone mass, such as one's race, body size, level of exercise, smoking, type of diet and/or hormonal activity. Daily physical activity and plenty of calcium are not only essential, but are also the most effective ways to minimize other harmful factors while keeping our bones strong.

Actual bone loss (when more bone is taken away than is formed) usually begins in the mid-40s and will occur in two phases. The slow phase of bone loss equally affects men and women and will continue throughout life. The accelerated phase of bone loss is limited to women and begins at menopause when women's bodies no longer produce estrogen. Certain drugs and/or medical conditions can also influence bone loss which puts both men and women at greater risk for osteoporosis.

Bone loss due to aging is also a function of your peak bone mass (how strong your bones were at their best) and age-related changes that will inevitably occur. For example, the body's ability to use Vitamin D changes and this vitamin is required by the body to absorb calcium. Finally, age-related bone loss is at its greatest in both women and men over the age of 70.

"New insights that control bone growth may soon lead to better therapies for this dangerous problem [bone loss]."

Science News, January 15, 2000

WHY WE LOSE
BONE MASS

SHORTAGE OF CALCIUM

One of the greatest risks to bone loss is the long-term shortage of dietary calcium. The skeleton is the largest storehouse of calcium in the body and calcium is necessary for many important biological functions including blood pressure regulation. It is important to know that the body adapts to shortages, and if our diet is low in calcium, our bodies will take the calcium they need for our heart and other organs from our bones. Needless to say, this risk increases for those who either avoid all dairy products for their fat content or have an intolerance to dairy products and do not eat other calcium-rich foods or supplements to meet their body's needs.

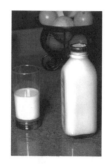

INACTIVE LIFESTYLE

A sedentary lifestyle or lack of exercise will also lead to bone loss. Weight-bearing activities, such as skipping or running, help our bones as they create mechanical stresses along the bones causing our body to respond by making our bones stronger. A very sedentary person is likely at greater risk of injury during frequent stresses, such as lifting a child, removing a turkey from the oven or shoveling snow. This is why it is important to increase physical activity in a safe way and learn proper body mechanics to reduce the risk of injury. Walking is a great way to introduce physical activity into your routine and is often the best exercise for inactive people or those with multiple health problems.

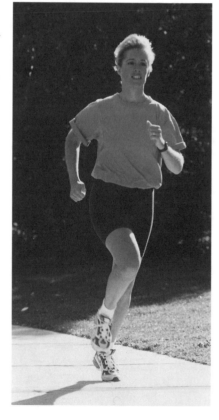

MENOPAUSE

The body stops producing estrogen at menopause and women therefore lose the protective effects it has on their bodies. At the same time, their body's rate of bone loss accelerates and their risk of heart disease increases. This accelerated rate of bone loss lasts for about ten to fifteen years, but after that, the overall rate of bone loss in women returns to the same rate as in men. For women, it is this accelerated phase of bone loss, combined with a lower average peak bone mass, that puts them at higher risk than men for osteoporosis and fractures.

Gather information to make an informed decision.

It has been shown that hormone replacement therapy can help reduce bone loss caused by hormone deficiency during menopause. And, while there are hormone-like products that have been shown to have positive estrogen-like effects on the bones and heart, while not appearing to increase the risk of breast cancer, it is very important to determine what is best for each person's specific needs. In addition to hormone replacement therapy, there are several medications which have been shown to partially restore lost bone and, more importantly, reduce the frequency of osteoporosis-related fractures. Discuss this issue with your doctor and learn the risks and benefits as they specifically relate to you so that you can make an informed decision. You may also want to contact the Osteoporosis Society of Canada (1-800-463-6842 or 1-416-696-2817), the National Osteoporosis Foundation in the United States (1-800-223-9994 or 1-202-223-2226), or an osteoporosis program in your community for more information.

FOOD FOR YOUR BONES

RECOMMENDED DAILY CALCIUM

AGE (years)	INTAKE (milligrams (mg))
4 to 8	800 mg
9 to 18	1300 mg
19 to 50	1000 mg
51+	1200* mg

*Higher intakes may be advisable if the risk of osteoporosis is high.

Calcium and Vitamin D recommendations are based on the 1997 Dietary Reference Intakes from the Institute of Medicine, Academy of Sciences. (study funded by the Food and Drug Administration, The U.S. Department of Agriculture, Health Canada and the U.S. National Institutes of Health)

Remember to drink lots of water every day.

CALCIUM & VITAMIN D INTAKE

Eating a well balanced diet with an emphasis on calcium, provides you with a solid base for healthy bones. Vitamin D, known as the sunshine vitamin (as your body produces it when exposed to the sun) helps your body absorb calcium. Milk is the best dietary source for helping bones as it is not only rich in calcium, but is also fortified with Vitamin D. Most North Americans can meet their Vitamin D requirements through milk, margarine and exposure to sunlight.

Our ability to metabolize nutrients, or absorb the good things from food, declines with age, and as a result, increases our risk of osteoporosis. This is why it is essential for elderly people to make every effort to maintain adequate amounts of Vitamin D and calcium in their diets. So, be sure to consult your doctor or dietitian if you believe you are not getting enough sun exposure or are unsure of your Vitamin D and/or calcium intakes.

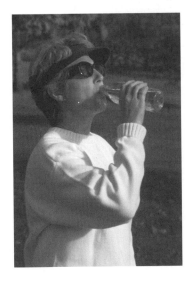

The recommended daily allowance of Vitamin D for adults is 300-400 international units (IU) and 600 IU for elderly people. Studies in nursing homes have shown that the overall hip fracture rate drops by 50 per cent when all residents are given supplements of 1000 mg of calcium and 1000 IU of Vitamin D.

Dairy products are the most calcium-rich foods available, and also contain many other nutrients essential to your health. While calcium is found in other foods, it is difficult to meet your daily calcium requirements through these sources alone. Plant foods are a less concentrated source of calcium than dairy products, and our bodies generally absorb only 30-50 per cent of the calcium contained in our diet. Cooked broccoli, Brussels sprouts, cauliflower, kale and rutabaga are your best plant food choices.

Calcium supplements should be taken with food to protect your stomach and improve absorption.

Preparation techniques, such as soaking beans or roasting nuts, can also increase the availability of calcium from these foods. Finally, there are some other plant foods that, although high in calcium, are not easily absorbed due to their high oxalate (oxalic acid salt) content. These include spinach, beet greens, Swiss chard and rhubarb. So compare your calcium sources and remember that all sources are not created equal. Consider one cup of 1% milk contains 314 mg of calcium of which 32 percent is absorbed (100.5 mg), versus one serving of broccoli (three spears) that contains 51 mg of calcium of which only 50 percent (25.5 mg) is absorbed.

CALCIUM & VITAMIN D INTAKE (cont'd)

Calcium supplements are a must if you are not able to meet your age group's recommended daily calcium intake through food, and if you have any doubts about the amount of calcium in your diet, consult your doctor or dietitian. Liquid calcium is available and can be easily added to soups and beverages. You can also use calcium-rich milk products in your baking and cooking, and if tofu is part of your diet, remember that either calcium or magnesium salt is used during its production. Firm tofu made with calcium is an excellent source of dietary calcium.

LACTOSE INTOLERANCE

Lactose is a natural sugar in all milk products and is normally digested easily in the body. People who have lactose intolerance cannot digest, or break down, this sugar properly and as a result, must often avoid milk or milk products. If you have lactose intolerance, consult your doctor or registered dietitian for calcium and milk alternatives. Many lactose intolerant people use tablets or drops that, when chewed after drinking/eating dairy products or added to regular milk, will help them digest lactose. These tablets and drops are available at most drugstores. Ready-to-use, lactose-reduced milk is also now available in most grocery stores.

PHOSPHORUS

Phosphorus is another important mineral for bone and tissue growth and is found in almost all foods, especially meat, fish, poultry, dairy products, eggs, peas, beans and nuts. North American adults usually take in twice the recommended dietary allowance in their diets and as a result, phosphorus deficiency is rare.

MAGNESIUM

Magnesium is needed in bone growth and in basic metabolic functions, and also helps the working of nerves and muscles. Magnesium is found in whole

A one cup serving of fortified orange juice contains approximately 300 mg of calcium.

grains, green leafy vegetables, nuts, beans, bananas, apricots, meat and milk. The recommended daily allowance of magnesium for adult women is 320 mg and 420 mg for men. Supplements are not usually required as we tend to take in enough magnesium through our diets and/or use of multi-vitamins.

SALT INTAKE

Eating large amounts of protein-rich foods, in combination with a low calcium intake can also lead to significant calcium loss. Salty foods also make your body lose calcium and as a result, most North Americans face this risk due to our high-salt diets. It is important to know that one teaspoon (2400 mg) of salt per day is more than adequate. Some simple ways to control your salt intake is to favor fresh vegetables, avoid fast foods and canned food and only add salt at the table and not during cooking.

MONITOR YOUR CAFFEINE & ALCOHOL INTAKE

Soya chips are available at most health food stores and provide a source for a calcium snack food.

People who ingest high amounts of caffeine from drinking a lot of coffee, tea or colas often lose more calcium than those who do not rely on caffeine. So try cutting down on, or eliminating, your caffeine intake by choosing to drink one of the many available decaffeinated coffees or teas instead. Heavy consumption of alcohol can also cause, or increase the risk of, osteoporosis even if you have no other risk factors.

NATURAL SOURCES OF CALCIUM

Following is a list of common foods with calcium content. Make a copy of this list and keep it on hand to help you plan your meals. The chart lists each calcium source with its corresponding calcium content in milligrams (mg). Total fat content in grams (g) has also been included for those who want to monitor their fat intake as well. Serving size is in metric with imperial equivalents and includes milliliters (mL), cups and tablespoons, grams (g) and ounces (oz).

FOOD FOR YOUR BONES

Dairy Products	Serving	Calcium Content (mg)	Fat Content (g)
Milk, whole	250 mL - 1 cup	308	9
Milk, 2%	250 mL - 1 cup	314	5
Milk, 1%	250 mL - 1 cup	317	3
Milk, skim	250 mL - 1 cup	319	trace
Milk, skim (added milk solids)	250 mL - 1 cup	372	1
Milk, chocolate, 2%	250 mL - 1 cup	300	5
Buttermilk	250 mL - 1 cup	301	2
Milk, Human	250 mL - 1 cup	84	11
Skim milk powder	125 mL - 1/2 cup	425	trace
Whole milk powder	125 mL - 1/2 cup	617	18
Chocolate milk, powder + 2%	250 mL - 1 cup	324	6
Chocolate milk, syrup + 2%	250 mL - 1 cup	321	5
Eggnog, 7%	250 mL - 1 cup	349	20
Instant breakfast powder + 2%	250 mL - 1 cup	566	5
Milk shake, chocolate	250 mL - 1 cup	279	6
Milk shake, vanilla	250 mL - 1 cup	309	6
Yogurt beverage	200 mL - 3/4 cup	220	2
Yogurt, fruit-bottom, 1-2%	175 g - 3/4 cup	214	3
Yogurt, fruit-bottom, less 1%	175 g - 3/4 cup	281	trace
Yogurt, plain, 1-2%	175 g - 3/4 cup	320	3
Yogurt, plain, greater 4%	175 g - 3/4 cup	264	10
Cheddar cheese (5 cm x 2cm x .5 cm/2 " x 3/4 " x 1/4 ")	4 slices - 52 g 1 - 3/4 oz	378	17
Cheddar, processed cheese (thin slices)	2 slices	239	10
Cheddar, processed cheese, light (thin slices)	2 slices	256	7
Processed Cheese Spread	50 mL - 1/4 cup	300	11
Cream cheese	50 mL - 1/4 cup	39	17
Swiss cheese (5 cm x 2cm x .5 cm/2 " x 3/4" x 1/4")	4 slices - 46 g 1 - 1/2 oz	438	13
Parmesan, grated	125 mL - 1/2 cup	727	16
Feta cheese	125 mL - 1/2 cup	403	17

Food Made With Dairy Products	Serving	Calcium Content (mg)	Fat Content (g)
Pudding, chocolate (ready to eat)	125 mL - 1/2 cup	124	6
Pudding, vanilla (ready to eat)	125 mL - 1/2 cup	105	4
Pizza, cheese, 1 medium	1/8 pizza	117	3
Nachos with cheese	(6-8) 113 g - 4 oz	272	19
Taco, fast food	1 small taco	221	21
Cheese Fondue	125 mL - 1/2 cup	541	15
Macaroni & cheese, (Kraft™ dinner)	250 mL - 1 cup	167	18
Pancake, plain, cooked (mix plus milk, egg, oil, 10 cm/4" diameter)	1 pancake	82	3
Pancake, whole-wheat, cooked (mix plus milk, egg, oil 10 cm/4" diameter)	1 pancake	110	3
Waffle, plain, frozen (ready-to-heat, 10 cm/4" dia.)	1 waffle	86	3
Cream of chicken soup (made with 2% milk)	250 mL - 1 cup	193	10
Cream of mushroom soup (made with 2% milk)	250 mL - 1 cup	192	13
Cream of tomato soup (made with 2% milk)	250 mL - 1 cup	172	5
Clam chowder, New England (made with 2% milk)	250 mL - 1 cup	201	5
Sauce, white, home-prepared (2% milk)	250 mL - 1 cup	312	28

FOOD FOR YOUR BONES

Other Food Sources	Serving	Calcium Content (mg)	Fat Content (g)
Molasses, blackstrap	15 mL - 1 tbsp	79	0
Sesame crunch (crisp)	4 pieces	247	12
Milk chocolate, plain, bars	1 bar - 50 g/1 3/4 oz	96	15
Coffee substitute Ovaltine™ (powder + milk)	250 mL - 1 cup	310	9
Sesame seeds (whole, dried)	15 mL - 1 tbsp	89	5
Baked beans, canned with pork	250 mL - 1 cup	163	4
Beans, navy, canned (solids and liquid)	250 mL - 1 cup	130	1
Beans, soybeans (dry, boiled)	250 mL - 1 cup	185	16
Beans, white, canned (solids and liquid)	250 mL - 1 cup	202	1
Tofu, firm (made with calcium)	60 mL - 1/4 cup	430	3
Tofu, firm (made with nigari)	60 mL - 1/4 cup	129	3
Tofu, regular (made with calcium)	60 mL - 1/4 cup	220	3
Tofu, regular (made with nigari)	60 mL - 1/4 cup	67	3
Almonds (dry roasted, salt added)	125 mL - 1/2 cup	206	38
Almonds (oil roasted)	125 mL - 1/2 cup	146	42
Sardine, Atlantic, canned (in oil, drained with bone,7.5 cm/3")	4 sardines 48 g - 3/4 oz	183	5
Salmon, Sockeye, canned (solids + bone + liquid-salt)	125mL - 1/2 cup	181	8
Pickerel / Walleye (baked/broiled)	1 fillet	175	2
Figs (dried, uncooked)	10 figs	269	2
Kale (cooked, boiled, drained)	125 mL - 1/2 cup	49	trace
Broccoli spears (boiled, drained)	3 spears	51	trace
Orange, raw	1 fruit	52	trace
Brussel sprouts (boiled, drained)	4 sprouts	30	trace
Cauliflower (raw)	250 mL - 1 cup	23	trace
Rutabaga (cubed, boiled, drained)	125 mL - 1/2 cup	43	trace

BENDING &
MUSCLE IMBALANCES

Your spine consists of your neck, mid-back, lower back, sacrum (triangular bone below your lower back) and tailbone. Jelly doughnut-like discs separate the bones in your neck, mid-back and lower back to allow for movement. The neck has a tremendous amount of rotation, or ability to turn, such as allowing you to safely look over your shoulder when either driving or riding a bike. And, since this rotation movement is small in the lower back, we often hear about lower back twisting-type injuries.

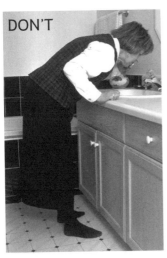

DON'T

We tend to develop habits where we either hold our spines in one position for long periods of time, such as sitting, or we repeatedly move in one direction while not moving in the opposite direction. This includes frequent forward bending at our lower backs during actions such as reaching in to the refrigerator, bending over a low sink to brush our teeth or tying a shoe.

DON'T

The most common excessive neck movements involve looking down to read, poking our heads forward during driving and sleeping with too many pillows. Over time, all of these actions can lead to a loss of neck mobility or movement. As a result, muscles shorten on one side of our spine and stretch or become longer on the opposite side. These muscle imbalances are often the cause of the bent forward postures we see in people with rounded shoulders, hunched shoulders or a loss of the natural inward curve in their lower back. Muscle imbalances also lead to long-term weaknesses and a reduced ability for the muscles to work as they should.

Most deformities in older adults are the visible effects of poor habits over many years but are, more

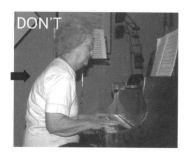

importantly, preventable. Simple efforts to regularly perform proper stretching, muscle-strengthening exercises and postural retraining will all work to correct these muscle imbalances.

COMPRESSIVE FORCES ON YOUR SPINE

Any time you move your body forward at the waist, your spine curves forward, and a force called a 'flexion moment' is put on your spine. Compression, or downward pressure through the spine, increases with these flexion moments and the disc compression that occurs during these movements is largely believed to be responsible for spinal injuries and fractures of the vertebrae (small bones) in your spine.

The least amount of compression in your spine occurs when you lie flat on your back. The amount of compression becomes greater whenever you either stand, sit or bend forward while standing or sitting. It is important to know that while improperly bending forward can put you at risk for injury, this movement puts those with osteoporosis at a much greater risk for spinal fracture.

Compression on your spine is least when you lie flat on your back.

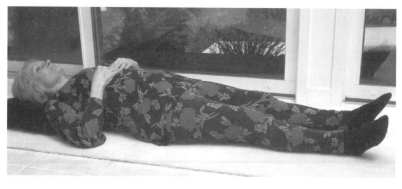

The amount of compression becomes greater whenever you bend forward in standing or sitting.

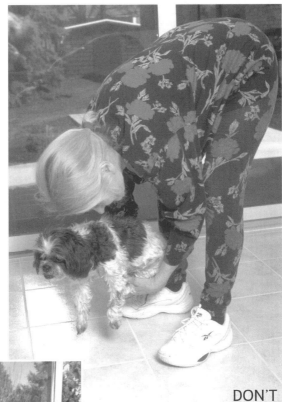

DON'T

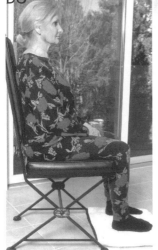

DO

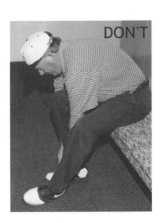

DON'T

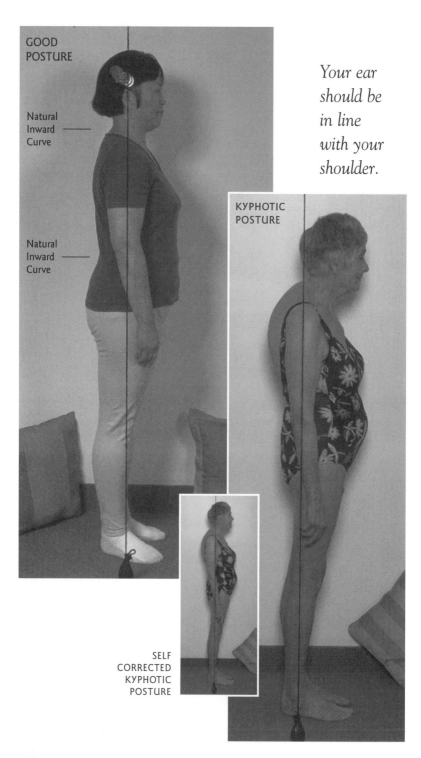

GOOD
POSTURE

Natural Inward Curve

Natural Inward Curve

Your ear should be in line with your shoulder.

KYPHOTIC POSTURE

SELF CORRECTED KYPHOTIC POSTURE

PLUMBLINE POSTURES

Your neck has a natural inward curve, or hollow, just above your shoulders. Proper standing posture is when your ears are in line with your shoulders. However it is very common for people to not know, or pay attention, to how they are standing, as they often carry their heads forward and away from their shoulders with their chins poking forward. Your lower back also has a natural inward curve and this hollow is also lost when your lower back is rounded from poor sitting postures or bending forward.

Forward bent posture can be caused by poor, long-standing habits and will increase the likelihood of muscle imbalances. However, these imbalances are correctable over time with proper stretching, strengthening and posture retraining.

A similar bent-forward posture can also be caused by a breakdown of the spine in people with osteoporosis and correction of bone changes, such as those that come with a spinal fracture, is not possible. However, muscle imbalances in people with osteoporosis can be targeted for stretching and strengthening to improve the person's overall posture and comfort. One way to help this problem is to stand tall, tuck in your stomach and occasionally shift your weight from one foot to the other during long periods of standing. You might also try resting one foot on an elevated surface (such as a step or bench) to ease the strain on your lower back during these times.

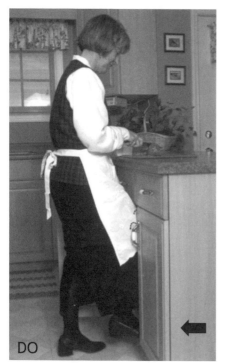

DO

← FOOT ELEVATED
TO EASE STRAIN
ON BACK

SIT SAFELY & PROTECT YOUR SPINE

You should also pay close attention to how you sit, for we now often sit for long periods of time while holding poor postures in harmful positions. When you sit, muscles that support your lower back will easily get tired. With muscle fatigue, the inward curve, or hollow in your lower back, is lost and you end up slouching. At the same time, muscles that support your head and neck also tire, and the inward curve in your neck is lost as you poke your head and neck forward. And once the slouched posture of your lower back takes over, it is next to impossible to maintain or regain good posture in your head, neck or upper spine.

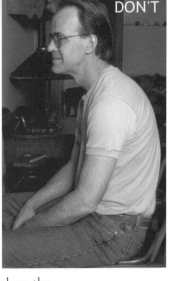

Unfortunately, we have many poor habits in our daily lives involving poor

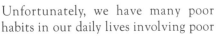

postures. We sit forward on the edge of our chair, hunched over, with our heads poked forward, while reading a book. Some of us lie on a couch or bed while leaning on one elbow (creating imbalances and a sideward curve of our spines). Many of us also hold our arms out, unsup-

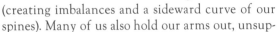

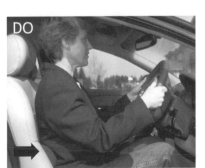

ported, while typing for many hours a day at work. All of these activities lead to the same results - headaches, sore necks, backs and shoulders, and additional pressures on our spines which, over the long term, can result in significant muscle imbalances and serious physical problems.

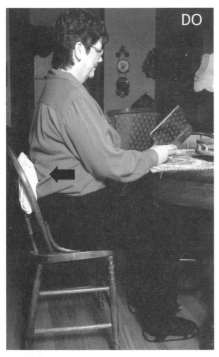

You should always try to use a lower backrest while sitting as most chairs do not provide sufficient lower back support. A lower back roll, or cylinder-shaped piece of foam, can be used in any chair, sofa, car or theater seat. Just tuck the roll into the small of your back at your waistline as you sit back. Lower back rolls come in various densities (hardness) of foam, so be sure you are comfortable with a roll before you buy it. There are also a variety of small pillows and full back supports available, and if you don't have such a support, try using a rolled-up towel instead.

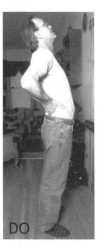

Healthy Hints

Travel smart:

- Be prepared to bring your own back support
- Give your body regular stretch breaks
- If it is not possible to stop and stretch on long trips, change your sitting position and stretch often to give your back relief
- Keep a back roll or small pillow in your car
- Try an adjustable full back support

SIT SAFELY & PROTECT YOUR SPINE

DESKWORK

Make sure your desk or computer chair has adequate support for your lower back, and if it does

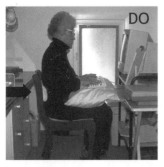

DO

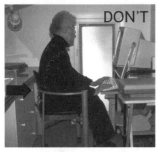

DON'T

not, be sure to add additional support. Try also to keep your feet flat on the floor or on a footrest as much as possible. When typing, keep your shoulders relaxed and your arms at your sides with your elbows bent at a 90-degree angle. Hold your forearms and wrists parallel to the floor. Sit about one arm's length from the screen, and position your monitor level with your eyes so that you can keep your head and neck relaxed and upright without straining.

Healthy Hints

User-friendly deskwork:

- Stretch every 60 minutes, or more often, if you feel strain
- Walk around every hour if possible
- Always hold the telephone receiver in your hand
- If you use the phone often, try a hands-free headset or speaker phone

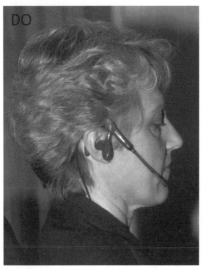

DO

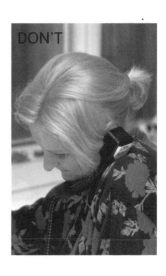

DON'T

SAFE &
HEALTHY DRIVING

While driving is one of our most common "sitting" activities, it is also one of the greatest causes for developing poor posture and muscle imbalances. And for those with weak bones or osteoporosis, a simple trip to the grocery store can result in significant neck and back pain or even a fracture.

All car seats are not created equal. Many driver's seats now have built-in and adjustable back (lumbar) supports. If you do not have an adjustable seat in your car, be sure to add support. When driving, position yourself from the steering wheel in a way that allows you to maintain an upright posture for both your head and neck. Place your hands on the steering wheel at the 9 and 3 o'clock positions with elbows slightly bent as you will find this allows you to keep your shoulders relaxed. Door or center console armrests should also be used as they increase your comfort while reducing neck and shoulder fatigue. Adjust rear-view mirrors so you do not have to lean forward or twist to view them. Finally, it is best to take a walking and stretch break every one or two hours during long trips, but if this is not possible, change your sitting position and stretch often to give your back relief.

GETTING IN AND OUT OF YOUR CAR

Getting in and out of the car can be difficult, especially for people with back pain or osteoporosis.

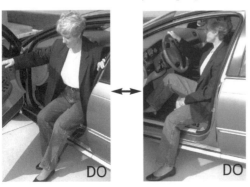

DO   DO

Sliding your car seat back prior to leaving your car is important as it gives you more room to get in and out. If your car seat is lower than your hip level when standing, it is best to get into your car backwards. Stand with your back towards the seat of your car and support

GETTING IN AND OUT OF YOUR CAR (cont'd)

yourself with both hands on the car. Keeping your back straight, bend at your hips and knees as you sit. Once sitting, pull in your stomach and then swing one leg in at a time.

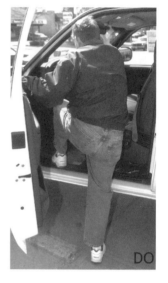

To get out of the car, go forward while supporting yourself. People with back pain usually try to keep their legs close together as they move in and out of the car, placing less rotary strain on their spines. But, remember that your legs are heavy and your back takes their weight when you lift them off the ground. Contracting your abdominal muscles also helps to reduce the strain on your back when you lift your legs off the ground. If the seat of your car is high, for instance as in sports utility vehicles or trucks, it is best to get in frontwards and get out backwards. This also works best if you have a step or running board on the truck. Remember to bend at the hips and knees, keep your back straight and your stomach pulled in tight. If you have arthritic joints and/or osteoporosis, get assistance when getting in and out of the car. While it sounds like a lot of effort and planning, injuries frequently occur when people get in and out of the car.

LIFTING ITEMS OUT OF YOUR CAR

Lifting heavy objects after a long time of sitting and driving is a high-risk situation for back injury. And, if you are at risk or have osteoporosis, the risk for injury is much greater. So, when you get out of the car, take a few minutes to move about and do a few back bends before unloading your car.

If the load you need to lift is manageable, remember to keep your spine straight, tuck your stomach in, and bend at the knees and hips. If you have items on

Always adjust your mirrors so you don't have to lean forward or twist to view them.

the passenger seat, get out of the car and walk around to unload them instead of trying to reach further into the car. If you have items on the back seat, do not twist and reach for them. Get out of the car first and then flip the front seat forward to give you enough space to position yourself properly before lifting.

Finally, the most difficult lifting occurs when getting objects from the trunk of a car. Remember that 10 pounds of potatoes or a case of pop are considered heavy objects, so take extra care when you are lifting them out of a deep trunk. Keep your back straight, your stomach pulled in, and bend forward at the hips before lifting, and if you can, avoid strenuous bending by lifting heavy objects in steps.

ONE FOOT ON GROUND LIFT: TRUNK OR BACK SEAT

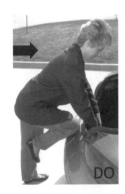

- Place one knee on car bumper or back seat with your standing leg slightly bent
- Keeping your back straight, bend at your hips and knees
- Slide the item close to you, look straight ahead, and lift with your legs while maintaining a straight back
- Always hold the item close to your body and turn by moving your feet instead of twisting your waist or back

TWO FEET ON GROUND LIFT: TRUNK OR BACK SEAT

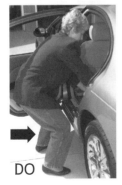

- Stand as close as possible to the car with your feet shoulder-width apart
- Keeping your back straight, lean forward by bending at your hips and knees
- Move item close and hold tight to your body, look straight ahead and return to an upright position by lifting with your legs

EVERYDAY LIFE ACTIVITIES

Maintaining good posture is important and especially during your many daily activities that place compression forces throughout your spine. Any time you bend forward, compression on your spine is higher and this action will put you at much greater risk of injury or a fracture if your bones are weak. If you have osteoporosis, you may want to consult a physical therapist/physiotherapist (PT) or occupational therapist (OT) to teach you how to safely perform everyday activities within your home.

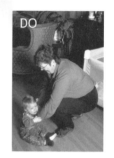

LIFTING

Remember that any form of lifting, either light or heavy, will always put compression forces on your spine and increase your risk of injury. And even during simple bending forward movements, compression forces increase as the entire weight of your torso, arms and head (about half your total body weight) are being held out and away from your body's centre of gravity. So, reduce your risks by following these lifting guidelines:

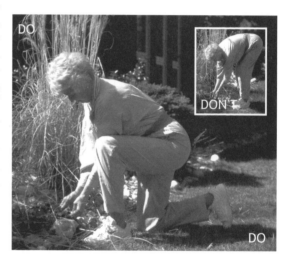

Lifting Guidelines

- Keep your back straight and abdominal muscles contracted
- Bend at your hips and knees
- Lift with your legs
- Do not lift anything heavy above your shoulder level
- Keep the item you are carrying close to your body
- Do not twist your back, move your feet to turn

LIFTING DURING HOUSEHOLD ACTIVITIES

So what does this mean in everyday home life?

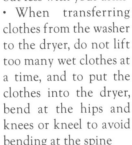
DO

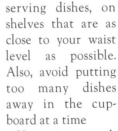
DO

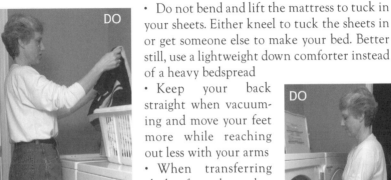

- Do not bend and lift the mattress to tuck in your sheets. Either kneel to tuck the sheets in or get someone else to make your bed. Better still, use a lightweight down comforter instead of a heavy bedspread
- Keep your back straight when vacuum- ing and move your feet more while reaching out less with your arms
- When transferring clothes from the washer to the dryer, do not lift too many wet clothes at a time, and to put the clothes into the dryer, bend at the hips and knees or kneel to avoid bending at the spine
- Store dishes, including heavier serving dishes, on shelves that are as close to your waist level as possible. Also, avoid putting too many dishes away in the cup- board at a time
- Heavy items, such as sugar or flour should be stored at waist level or in can- isters on the counter
- Store spices and other small, light items, such as tea or pasta, on the higher shelves

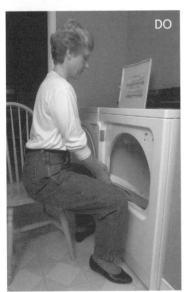
DO

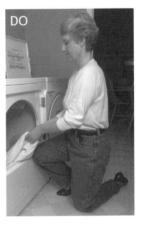
DO

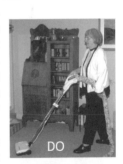
DON'T

EVERYDAY LIFE ACTIVITIES

SHOVELING AND SNOW REMOVAL

Shoveling snow is very hard work and requires heavy lifting and walking on often-slippery surfaces which increases one's risk of falling. Statistics show that the first big snowfall is usually accompanied by an increase in lower back injuries and heart attacks. While the safest way is to have someone else shovel snow for you, if you need to shovel, take the necessary steps before starting.

Like any significant exercise, shoveling snow requires a warm-up, good body mechanics and movements and is finished with a cool-down period. Keeping your back straight, bending at the hips and knees and moving your feet rather than twisting your back are all very important. Finally, using a snow scoop can also help reduce the strain shoveling and lifting will put on your back.

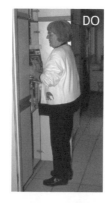

DO

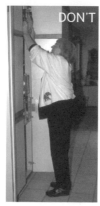

DON'T

PURSES & CARRY BAGS

Most women carry a purse every day. Purses should be light and tucked under the arm. Shoulder straps

CARRY BAG HANDLE

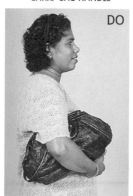

DO

should be worn across the body and not hung from one shoulder as carrying heavy loads over your shoulder can lead to many physical problems. A fanny pack, or a small, light purse with a shoulder strap is preferred. Backpack style purses are also helpful, provided the load remains light and you carry the bag with good posture. For men, carrying a wallet in the same back pocket may be convenient but can also contribute to back problems later in life.

You should also avoid the common mistake of carrying several

If you have osteoporosis, do not lift anything more than 2 pounds (1 kg) above your shoulders.

bags of groceries in one hand just to save time, as this will also increase your risk of injury. And when you travel, be kind to your back by using small suitcases (to reduce the likelihood that they will be heavy) and choose suitcases with wheels and push-pull handles for easier use.

Healthy Hints

- Use a small purse or fanny pack
- Carry your purse tucked under your arm and be sure to alternate sides while carrying it
- Keep your elbows slightly bent when carrying briefcases, suitcases and groceries
- Choose small to medium-sized luggage with wheels and a pull-push handle
- Use a carry bag handle to spread the load when carrying one or more plastic, cloth or string bags
- Two lighter loads are better than one heavy load

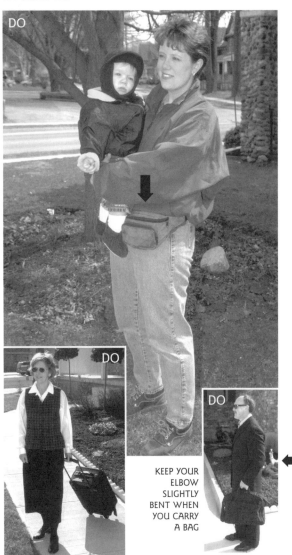

DO

DO

DO

KEEP YOUR ELBOW SLIGHTLY BENT WHEN YOU CARRY A BAG

MEDICINE FOR YOUR BONES

There is a wonderful medicine that helps build and maintain strong bones, improves cardiovascular fitness and keeps muscles strong. It improves balance, prevents falls and decreases blood cholesterol. It reduces risk of heart disease, heart attack and diabetes. This medicine improves glucose control in people who are diabetic, helps with weight loss and improves functional independence. What is this miracle medicine? It is exercise!

Many people enjoy exercise but more of us do not. While exercise can be fun, it does not have to be fun in order to be effective for our bodies. Brushing teeth, flossing or taking medication or vitamins are not fun activities. Eating enough roughage, maintaining a low fat diet and low sweet intake are not fun, yet we do all of these things to maintain our body and to stay healthy. The same goes for exercise; while we do not have to enjoy exercise, it is an essential part of a healthy lifestyle and helps reduce the risk of diseases such as osteoporosis.

You are lucky if you enjoy exercise but if you do not, you will have to be creative to fit exercise into your lifestyle. Think of activities that will not take too much time, will not interfere with what you like to do and are feasible for you to continue for the rest of your life. If you have a condition that prevents you from exercising, talk to your doctor or consult a physiotherapist as there are safe exercises available for everyone. And, if you develop any joint pain or other problems after beginning exercise, see your doctor or physiotherapist right away.

Regular exercise will not always be boring. Once you start feeling its benefits you will make it a regular habit. You will begin to notice that your neck, back or joint problems do not bother you as much when you are exercising and you will find that you have more strength and endurance to do the many things you like to do, such as shopping, gardening, playing cards or going dancing.

Exercise regularly to keep a lean body, maintain muscle mass, flexibility, strong bones and a healthy heart and lungs.

WHY WE NEED TO EXERCISE

- Improve bone mass and prevent bone loss associated with inactivity
- Improve the effect of medicines designed to improve bone mass
- Improve muscle strength (muscle mass is lost as early as age 30)
- Improve balance and coordination
- Improve flexibility and prevent/correct muscle imbalances
- Improve heart and lung fitness
- Strengthen postural muscles and maintain an upright posture
- Reduce the risk of fracture
- Reduce pain (circulation and joint lubrication improves/brain produces painkillers)
- Improve overall mobility, functional independence and quality of life

YEAR-ROUND EXERCISE

Exercise is the recurring theme behind the prevention of many key diseases.

We lose muscle mass, become less flexible and have less stamina as we age. Many of us don't recognize that we have become less fit and less healthy until we notice a significant physical problem. Yet regular exercise is key to feeling better and having a healthy life. A year-round exercise program should consist of stretching exercises, strengthening exercises for your muscles and your bones and physical activity for your heart and lungs (cardiovascular exercise). If you have not exercised previously you must remember to start off slowly and gradually increase the intensity of your program. Always prepare your body before exercising through warm-ups and cool-downs regardless of the exercise, whether it be sports like tennis, running or cycling, or housework, such as raking leaves or shoveling snow.

A three-to five-minute warm-up prepares your body and muscles for your workout. Mimicking your chosen activity at an easy pace is also a good way to warm

MEDICINE FOR
YOUR BONES

YEAR-ROUND EXERCISE (cont'd)

up as it will increase the circulation to the muscles
that you will soon be using more intensely. You
should slow your exercise to a gradual stop and then
take about five final minutes to cool down.

STRENGTHENING

Medical and physiotherapy experts now know that

while we all lose muscle mass at
an early age, we can also work to
reverse or slow this process. So
begin regular exercise to first
develop your muscle strength
and then to increase the
endurance of your muscles.
Muscle strength is the power
that your muscles have and muscle endurance is the ability of
your muscles to work for long
periods of time without fatigue.

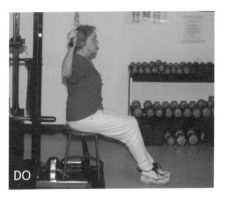

Vigorous strength training can be dangerous if
you either have weak bones, use poor technique or

have never performed these
exercises before. If you have
osteoporosis or low bone mass,
avoid lifting weights that put
your body in a forward bent
position for this increases compression forces on the spine
and increases risk of fracture.
If you are unsure, consult your
doctor and/or physiotherapist
before you begin a strengthening program. Try to do your
strengthening or weight train-

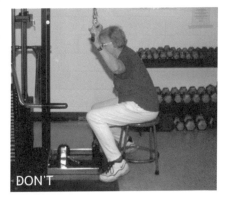

ing with function in mind. In other words, think
about how your muscles work during specific
activities you perform on a regular basis or during
your sports and recreational activities.

Always maintain good posture and make sure the weights are not extended more than about 30 degrees from your body. Keep your abdominal muscles contracted, your back straight and your knees unlocked. It is especially important to do hip strengthening in a standing position as hips need to be strong and developed to support your body during most daily activities. You can do weight training in your home or at a gym. While free weights, dumbbells and exercise machines are common, you can also use your own body weight as resistance weight training with such exercises as push-ups or semi-squats. Other weight training tools can include soup cans, books and specialty strengthening latex bands or tubing.

It is also important to know that weight training and resistive exercises should not be done every day. For when you train, tiny tears occur in the muscles and your muscles need a certain amount of time to repair themselves. It is better to weight train two or three times per week with at least one day of rest between each session.

Strengthening Guidelines (Arms & Legs)

- Always lift and lower the weight in a slow and controlled fashion
- When exercising a specific muscle group, your goal is to fatigue or tire that muscle group. This means lifting until your muscle(s) feel too tired to lift the weight even once more. At this point you need to rest that muscle group
- For strength training, the weight or resistance is correct if your muscle is tired after one set of 8-12 repetitions of the exercise. Rest and repeat repetitions for one or two more sets
- For muscle endurance training, the weight or resistance is correct if your muscle is tired after one set of 20 repetitions of the exercise. Rest and repeat 20 repetitions for two more sets
- Exercises should not be painful while you perform them or lead to excessive soreness afterwards

N.B. Opinion varies on the need to repeat sets of repetitions in strength training. Some believe one set is adequate so choose what works best for you.

FLEXIBILITY & STRETCHING

We inevitably lose muscle flexibility over time from inactivity and poor habits. The imbalances associated with lost flexibility often lead to pain and interfere with our movement. To improve or increase flexibility, you should perform stretching exercises every day. Once you have regained your flexibility, stretching every other day will be enough to maintain these gains. Always remember to take a few minutes to warm your muscles up before your stretches. This can be done by simple walking, jogging on the spot or, if you prefer, by taking a warm shower.

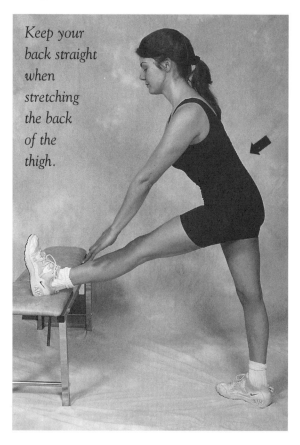

Keep your back straight when stretching the back of the thigh.

Stretching Guidelines

- Move in the stretch to the point where you feel a comfortable pull in the muscle; if this pull lessens during the stretch, stretch a little more. You should never feel pain during stretching
- For optimal results, hold each stretch for 30 seconds and if you are unable to hold it for that long, maintain the stretch as long as possible. Return to the start position between each stretch
- Always stretch both sides of each muscle group (i.e. left and right side of neck)
- Repeat each stretch 3 times

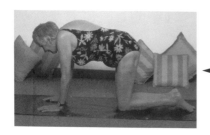 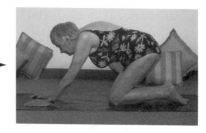

MAINTAIN THE FLEXIBILITY IN YOUR HIPS

HEART & LUNG FITNESS

Aerobic or cardiovascular exercises involve whole body activity as you use all of your large muscle groups while walking, jogging, cycling or swimming. Aerobic exercises are exercises that safely and comfortably increase your breathing and heart rates for an extended period of time without disturbing the balance between your intake and use of oxygen. Start aerobic exercise slowly and gradually increase both the duration and intensity of the exercise over time. You might also want to vary the exercises for variety, but always monitor your pulse and listen to your body during vigorous exercise. Get ready to feel good, have more energy and exercise longer!

Drink lots of water prior to, during and after all exercise.

SWIMMING

Swimming and aquatic exercises are good forms of general exercise because they strengthen muscles, improve heart and lung fitness and are easy on the body's joints. However, because swimming and aquatic exercises are non-weight bearing, they have little if any beneficial effect on bone strengthening so if your chosen activity is swimming, you must also include weight-bearing exercises to strengthen your bones.

LET'S WALK FOR THE HEALTH OF IT

There is little scientific evidence to support walking as an activity that helps build or strengthen bones. However, it is obvious that walking is better than no activity as it provides many other benefits to your overall fitness and health.

For walking to be effective, it has to be based on the overload principle. In other words, you have to walk at a much faster pace than you usually would in order to gain the health benefits to your body including the strength of your bones. Walking has to be brisk, done regularly (three to four times per week) and for at least 30-60 minutes. This form of walking does not include walking with a toddler, shopping or pushing a stroller; nor does walking the dog count unless you walk vigorously for at least 30 minutes.

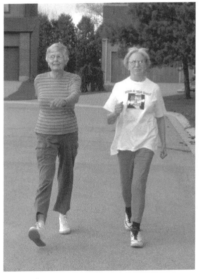

When you are walking you should be able to talk but not be able to carry on a normal conversation at the same time. You are working too hard, however, if you can only gasp out single words or manage the occasional grunt. Finally, using hand, wrist or ankle weights while walking is not recommended as they put too much added stress on your joints.

If your back hurts or you feel worn out, start with a shorter walk.

WALKING PROGRAM

If you have any concerns about your health or fitness, consult your doctor before starting a walking program. Professional help from a physiotherapist, kinesiologist or qualified personal trainer is also available.

When you first begin your walking program, start slowly with a five minute or less effort depending on your condition, and to avoid injuries or discourage-

LET'S TRY RUNNING

Running has become a popular form of exercise. Many people, even those who did not run when they were younger, are now starting to run in their 40s and 50s. Running can be safe for people with low bone mass as long as it is done under the supervision of a physiotherapist, for with their guidance, safety, posture, muscle imbalances and pain issues can all be addressed as they arise. You can start with five, 10-second intervals of running separated by 5-minute walks. Work up through a very gradual progression over five to six months until you are running 4- or 5-minute intervals separated by 1- to 2-minute walks. Eventually you can work up to 30- to 50-minute runs with 10-minute intervals of jogging, alternating with one to two minutes walking. The walking breaks are important for recovery and to prevent injury to your muscles and joints. If you have any questions about good running technique, take a "Learn to Run" course. These courses are usually advertised through either running equipment stores or running clubs.

Remember to do the talk test to determine how hard you are working.

WALK RUN PROGRESSION

The following twenty-week Walk Run Progression Table will help you work from initial 5-minute walks separated by 10-second runs through to 50 minutes of 10-minute runs separated by 2-minute walks. If you find, however, that the progression is too fast, stay at the previous week's schedule for two or three more weeks. Listen to your body. Success depends on gradual progression, taking your walk breaks and solving every muscle or joint problem as it arises. Use a stopwatch to time your intervals and keep a journal to track how far and long you run. Your speed should be slow at first and can gradually increase as you are comfortable. You should be able to talk but not be able to carry on a normal conversation at the same time. The figures in the table below represent minutes except where seconds (sec) are specified.

WALK RUN PROGRESSION
(minutes)

Week	Walk	Run	Walk	Run	Walk	Run	Walk	Run	Walk
1	5	10 sec	5	10 sec	5	10 sec	5	10 sec	5
2	5	20 sec	5	20 sec	5	20 sec	5	20 sec	5
3	5	30 sec	5	30 sec	5	30 sec	5	30 sec	5
4	5	30 sec	5	1	5	1	5	30 sec	5
5	5	1	5	1	5	1	5	1	5
6	5	1	4	2	4	2	4	1	5
7	5	2	4	2	4	2	4	2	5
8	5	2	3	3	3	3	3	2	5
9	3	3	2	3	2	3	2	3	5
10	3	3	2	4	2	4	2	3	5
11	3	4	2	4	2	4	2	4	5
12	2	5	2	5	2	5	2	5	5
13	2	5	2	6	2	6	2	5	5
14	2	6	2	7	2	7	2	6	5
15	2	6	2	7	2	7	2	6	5
16	2	7	2	8	2	8	2	7	5
17	2	8	2	8	2	8	2	8	5
18	2	8	2	9	2	10	2	8	5
19	2	9	2	10	2	10	2	9	5
20	2	10	2	10	2	10	2	10	5

- **Walk** means moderate to brisk walking pace
- **Run** means slow, moderate or fast jog, never a sprint
- **Remember** to do the talk test to determine how hard you are working

POSTURAL RETRAINING: EASY STEPS TO STRAIGHTEN UP

To be able to maintain good posture you need to be able to straighten your back, pull your shoulders back and tuck your stomach in. Sounds just like what your mother told you to do when you were a teen! You also need to be able to keep your back straight and stomach in while you are doing various activities - especially lifting and carrying activities that load more weight during the spine's movements.

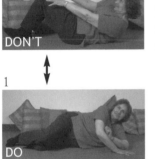

Postural retraining exercises are divided into four main sections. Some of the individual exercises have levels of increasing difficulty. You should progress through the levels at your own speed so that you are working on only one of the levels of a specific exercise at any one time. Since some exercises are done on the floor, you should take extra caution while getting up and down from the floor safely.

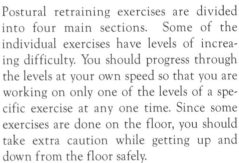

GETTING UP & DOWN FROM THE FLOOR

1) Roll onto your side and push yourself up into side sitting, never straight up.
2) Slowly move onto your hands and knees, place your hands on a chair or other solid object
3) Put one foot up and then the other; raise yourself into standing position

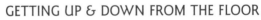

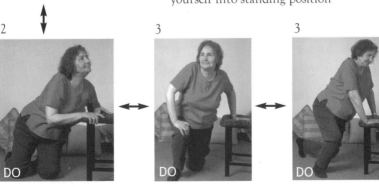

STATIC & DYNAMIC POSTURAL CORRECTION

The following postural correction exercises target the abdominal, shoulder and back muscles and should be done every day. Most of these exercises can be done just about anywhere. You may wish to try some of these exercises while waiting in queues at the bank, at the grocery store checkout or when sitting in a car during slow traffic.

STANDING POSTURAL CORRECTION

- Stand tall, straighten your spine, keep your head up and look straight ahead
- Roll your shoulders back, squeeze your shoulder blades together, then relax about ten percent
- Pull your stomach in by pulling your navel towards your backbone; maintain position
- Breathe deeply in and out ten times; relax

STANDING POSTURAL CORRECTION AT THE WALL

- Stand with your heels two to three inches away from the wall with your back against the wall. Place a small folded towel behind your lower back to fill the gap
- Straighten up, pull your shoulders back and your stomach in. With your back flattened against the wall breathe deeply in and out
Start with one minute and work up to five

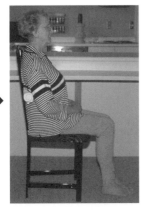

SITTING POSTURAL CORRECTION
* Sit right to the back of a straight-backed chair
* Sit up straight, look straight ahead, pull your shoulders back and stomach in
* Breathe deeply in and out in the corrected posture for one minute; relax

Repeat five times

This will help you maintain good posture while performing activities. You can progress this exercise by increasing the distance that you walk or try using your arms as you balance the box.

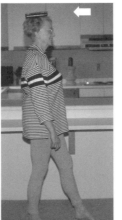

DYNAMIC POSTURAL CORRECTION
* Do the standing postural correction exercise
* Place a light paperback book or box of tissues on your head. Walk across the room; remove the book or box and relax

SITTING TALL WITH BOOK
* Do the sitting postural correction exercise (above) and maintain this posture. Place a light paperback book or box of tissues on your head
* Sit in your usual chair to watch TV, read a book or relax. Remain for five minutes, remove the book or box and relax

Repeat three to five times

ABDOMINAL STRENGTHENING

When performing a tummy tuck, do not allow your back to arch. If you cannot keep your back flat against the floor, the level of tummy tuck is too difficult for you to perform. Move up through the numbered levels of tummy tuck exercises as your strength permits. Work on one level at any one given time. As you become stronger and more skilled at a specific level, it's time to move onto the next level.

TUMMY TUCK
* Lie on the floor on your back, knees bent, feet flat. Pull your tummy in by pulling your navel up towards your ribs and in towards your backbone
* Feel your back flatten against the floor; your buttocks should not come up off the floor. Hold for ten counts, keep breathing; relax
Repeat five times

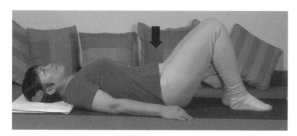

TUMMY TUCK WITH LEG SLIDE
* Perform and maintain tummy tuck (above)
* Slide one foot down along the floor until your leg is straight and resting on the floor
* Now slide the same leg back up to the starting position; relax. Alternate legs
Repeat five times with each leg

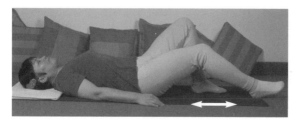

ABDOMINAL STRENGTHENING

TUMMY TUCK WITH FOOT LIFT: LEVEL 1

* Perform and maintain tummy tuck

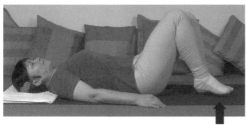

* Lift one foot a few inches off the floor
* Hold position for five counts, slowly lower foot, relax. Alternate sides
Repeat ten times with each leg

TUMMY TUCK WITH FOOT LIFT: LEVEL 2

* Perform and maintain tummy tuck
* Lift your left foot off the floor while bringing your

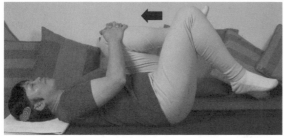

knee to your chest. Hold the top of your left knee with both hands
* Lift your right foot a few inches off the floor and hold this for five counts. Lower your right foot to the floor, then your left foot; relax. Alternate sides

Repeat ten times with each leg

TUMMY TUCK WITH FOOT LIFT: LEVEL 3

* Perform and maintain tummy tuck

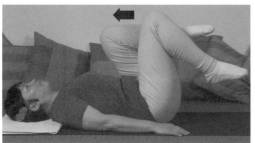

* Lift your left foot off the floor while bringing your knee to your chest
* Lift your right foot off the floor and bring your right leg up beside your left leg
* Lower your right foot slowly to the floor, then your left foot; relax. Alternate sides

Repeat ten times with each leg

ABDOMINAL STRENGTHENING

TUMMY TUCK WITH FOOT LIFT: LEVEL 4
* Perform and maintain tummy tuck
* Lift your right foot off the floor while bending 90 degrees at your hip
* Lift your left foot off the floor and bring it up beside your right leg
* Lower your left foot slowly to the floor, then your right foot; relax. Alternate sides

Repeat ten times with each leg

Don't hold your breath when performing Tummy Tuck exercises.

STAND TALL TUMMY TUCKS WITH LEG SLIDES
* Stand with your heels two to three inches away from, and your back against, a wall. Place a small folded towel behind your lower back to fill the gap
* Straighten up, pull your shoulders back, perform tummy tuck and hold
1. Slide one leg out to your side and move back slowly five times
2. Slide the same leg out to the front and move back slowly five times; relax

Repeat once on the other side

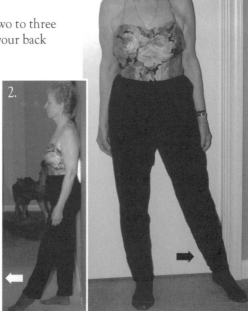

THE ABDOMINAL & BREATHING MUSCLE CONNECTION

One important segment of the abdominal muscle group has been found to work in cooperation with the diaphragm - our primary muscle for breathing, therefore, diaphragmatic breathing exercises are very beneficial. It has been found that the diaphragm not only controls breathing, but assists in stabilizing the spine. Diaphragmatic breathing can be done anywhere. When performed on a hard surface such as the floor, you get the benefit of a good spinal stretch.

DIAPHRAGMATIC BREATHING
* Lie on your back in a comfortable position
* You may have your knees bent or straight, and you may add a pillow to support your knees
* Place a box of tissues or a book on your abdomen just below the ribs
* Breathe in deeply through your nose; the box/book should rise. Breathe out through your mouth; the box/book should lower

Continue this relaxed breathing for five to ten minutes. Progress by contracting your abdominal muscles at the same time

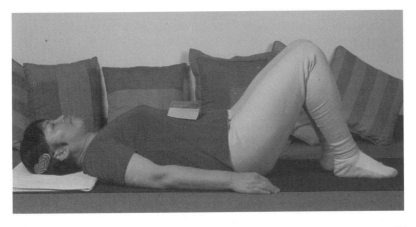

BACK STRAIGHTENING & STRENGTHENING

SITTING ARM RAISES

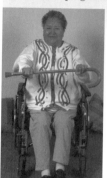

* Sit upright in a straight-backed chair, with your feet flat and look straight ahead. Pull your shoulders back, your stomach in and do not arch your lower back
* Hold a bar a shoulder width apart, palms down and elbows straight. Lift the bar as high as you can
* Breathe in as you lift, and out as you lower the bar

Repeat ten times

A broom handle, a roll from gift wrap or a cane makes a great bar for Arm Raises.

STANDING ARM RAISES

* Stand with your heels two to three inches away from, and your back against, a wall. Place a small folded towel behind your lower back to fill the gap
* Straighten up, pull your shoulders back and stomach in to flatten your back against the wall
* Holding a bar a shoulder width apart, palms down and elbows straight, lift the bar as high as you can
* Breathe in as you lift, and out as you lower the bar

Repeat ten times

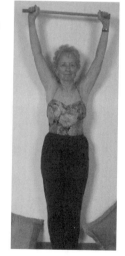

LYING ON STOMACH (PRONE LYING)

* Lie on your stomach, hands at your sides. Place one or more pillows under your stomach for comfort (if needed)
* Place a rolled towel under your forehead or turn your head to the side. Relax and breathe normally; you should feel comfortable

Start with one to five minutes and gradually increase to twenty minutes a day

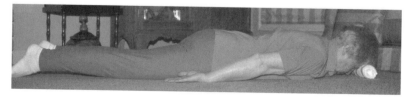

BACK STRAIGHTENING
& STRENGTHENING

PRONE LYING ON FOREARMS (THE SPHINX)

* Lie on your stomach for a few minutes to start
* Place your hands on the floor in front of you so that your elbows are bent at 90 degrees. Push up onto your elbows so your elbows are under your shoulders and your forearms and hands rest on the floor in front of you. Your hips and stomach should remain on the floor

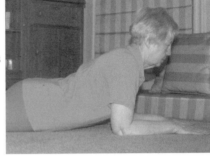

* Hold position for one minute, lower yourself and relax

Repeat five times; gradually increase the time you can hold this position to ten to fifteen minutes

Healthy Hints

If you have not been able to lie on your stomach for a long time or cannot seem to get comfortable, consult with a physiotherapist who can teach you how to attain this position. The position is used as a stretch and for exercises only

OPPOSITE ARM & LEG LIFTS

* Lie on your stomach with a towel roll under your forehead. Place your arms over your head with your elbows straight and thumbs pointing to the ceiling
* Hold your stomach in, squeeze your buttocks tight. Lift one arm and the opposite leg off the floor, hold five counts; relax. Alternate sides

Repeat ten times each

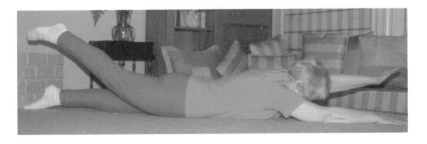

BACK STRAIGHTENING
& STRENGTHENING

BACKUPS: LEVEL 1
- Lie on your stomach with your hands behind your back or at your sides
- Hold your stomach in, squeeze your buttocks tight, hold ten counts; relax

Repeat ten times, progress through levels

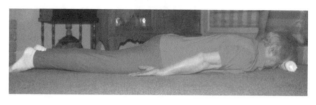

For comfort, pillow(s) can be placed under your abdomen for backup exercises.

LEVEL 2

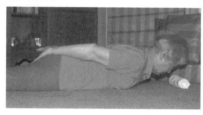

Lift your head and shoulders one to two inches off the floor

LEVEL 3

Lift your head and shoulders off the floor as high as you can

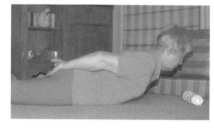

LEVEL 4

With your hands at your temples, lift your head and shoulders off the floor as high as you can

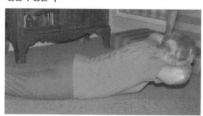

SHOULDER STRAIGHTENING & STRENGTHENING

STANDING SHOULDER-BLADE SQUEEZES:
POSITION 1
* Stand up straight with your feet a shoulder's width apart, knees slightly bent. Place your hands behind your back at the level of your pelvis
* Squeeze your shoulder blades together, hold three counts; relax

Repeat ten times

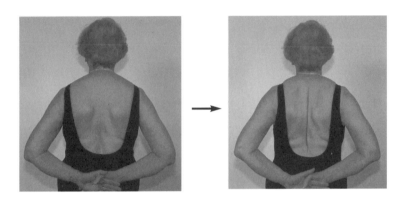

Place your hands at your waist for Position 2, behind your upper back for Position 3 and behind your temples for Position 4. If you experience pain or difficulty, consult a physiotherapist

POSITION 2	POSITION 3	POSITION 4

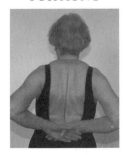 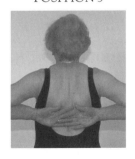 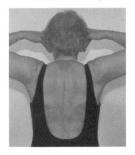

SHOULDER STRAIGHTENING & STRENGTHENING

LYING SHOULDER-BLADE SQUEEZES: POSITION 1
* Lie on your back, place your arms at your sides, bend your elbows to 90 degrees
* Push your elbows into the floor, squeeze your shoulder blades together, hold for five counts

Repeat ten times

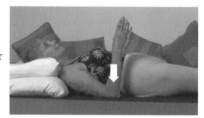

LYING SHOULDER-BLADE SQUEEZES: POSITION 2
* Lie on your back, place your arms at 90 degrees out to the side, bend your elbows to 90 degrees
* Push your elbows into the floor, squeeze your shoulder blades together, hold for five counts

Repeat ten times

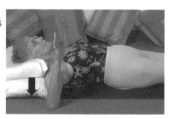

LYING SHOULDER-BLADE SQUEEZES: POSITION 3
* Lie on your back, place your arms at your sides, with your hands at your temples
* Push your elbows into the floor, squeeze your shoulder blades together, hold for five counts

Repeat ten times

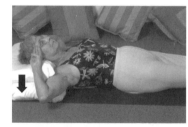

THE CROSS
* Lie on your stomach with a towel roll under your forehead. Place your arms stretched out to the sides at 90 degrees like a cross. Hold your stomach in and squeeze your buttocks tight
* Thumbs pointing to the ceiling, raise your arms from the floor, then slowly lower them

Repeat ten times, progress this exercise by holding small weights

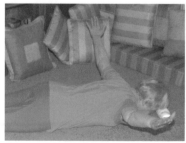

THE BIG V
* Stand facing the wall with your toes touching it
* Form a "V" with your arms, your hands touching the wall, while keeping your elbows straight. Tighten your stomach and do not arch your lower back
* Lift one arm away from the wall, return it, keep the "V", don't twist your body. Alternate sides

Repeat five to ten times; can also be performed lying on your stomach

Turn the palms of your hands towards your body, away from the wall or floor, prior to lifting your arms.

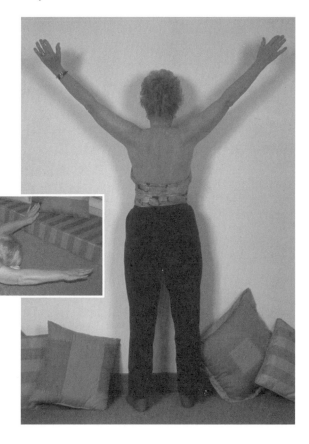

KEEPING YOUR BALANCE

TAI CHI

Good balance is important to prevent falls but it also becomes less stable as we get older. A person with low bone density is much more likely to fracture if they fall than is a person with normal bone density. The Chinese martial art of Tai Chi has been shown to be a very good way to strengthen muscles while improving balance. It has been shown to reduce incidents of falling in randomized controlled study trials. While many community and seniors' centers now offer Tai Chi programs, it is good to "shop around" before joining a Tai Chi program. Ask about the instructor's qualifications and how many movements are covered. There should be a minimum of ten movements and an instructor should be able to name each of them. If these questions cannot be answered, the program may not be either authentic or the right program for you.

BALANCE EXERCISES

Balance exercises are good to do as they challenge your ability to maintain balance and therefore increase your muscles ability to handle quick or unbalanced movements in your daily life. Following are balance exercises that will help you strengthen your legs as well as other balancing muscles. Many of these exercises can be performed anywhere and the more often you do them, the better. You may want to try these exercises while you are at the kitchen sink, at a bus stop or waiting for an elevator.

But remember, when your balance is challenged you are at increased risk of falling. That is why it is important to observe safety precautions when doing any type of balance training. Make sure that you stand near a solid object (counter, post or doorway) so that you can hold onto something if the need arises. These exercises require concentration so you may want to put your dog or cat in another room or take the phone off the hook to avoid being startled. Make sure you exercise on a bare, dry floor and remove all clutter from the area.

When performing walking balance exercises watch for hazards such as a change from carpet to flooring.

TOE RISES, BOTH FEET: LEVEL 1

* Stand at the kitchen counter, stand straight, hold on with both hands. Pull your stomach in and rise up on your toes as high as you can. Hold for five counts, slowly lower back down
Repeat this exercise ten times

Progress to holding on with one hand for Level 2, no hands for Level 3 and to raising both arms above your head for Level 4

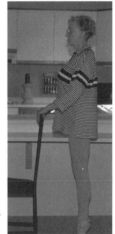

TOE RISES, ONE FOOT: LEVEL 1

* Hold onto counter with both hands and rise up on one foot. Hold this for five counts, slowly lower back down.
Alternate feet
Repeat this exercise ten times each side

Progress to holding on with one hand for Level 2, no hands for Level 3 and to raising both arms above your head for Level 4

TOE WALKING: LEVEL 1

Start toe walking once you reach Level 3 toe rises.

* Stand sideways at the counter, hold on with one hand. Stand tall, pull your stomach in, rise up on toes, walk forward ten steps. Walk backwards ten steps and lower back down
Repeat this exercise five times

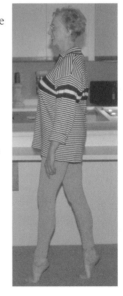

Progress to holding on only if needed for Level 2 and to walking around the house for Level 3

TANDEM WALKING: LEVEL 1

* Stand sideways at the counter holding on with one hand. Stand tall, pull your stomach in, walk forward heel to toe ten steps and back

Repeat this exercise five times

Progress to holding on only if needed for Level 2 and to walking around the house for Level 3

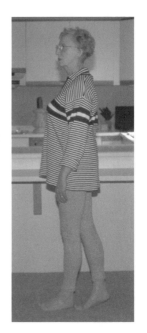

The next two balance exercises require a piece of elastic resistance band or tubing. These are available at most medical supply and exercise equipment stores. They come in different colors representing graded levels of difficulty. Start with the lowest resistance.

RESISTED WALKING SIDEWAYS : LEVEL 1

* Tie the band or tube around your legs just above your knees. Stand facing the counter holding on with both hands
* Stand tall, pull your stomach in, keep your toes pointing forward. Walk sideways ten steps and back to your starting position

Repeat this exercise five times, progress to holding on only if needed for Level 2

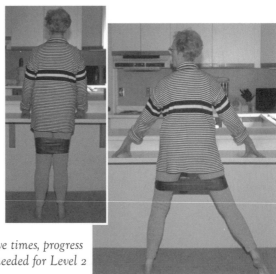

RESISTED WALKING FORWARD : LEVEL 1

* Tie the band or tube around your legs just above your knees. Stand sideways at the counter holding on with one hand
* Stand tall, pull tummy in, walk forward ten steps and back keeping band taut

Repeat this exercise five times, progress to holding on only if needed for Level 2

Walking on your heels is another good balance exercise.

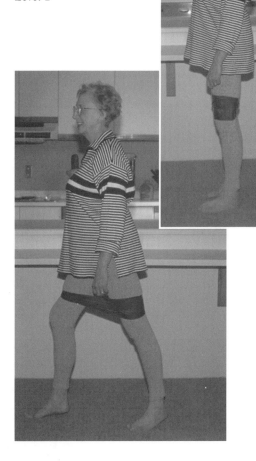

SPORTS & RECREATION

HIGH-RISK ACTIVITIES

Some sports are not recommended for people with osteoporosis. This is especially true for sports with a high risk of falling such as skiing, skating or rollerblading. Contact sports such as hockey are not recommended either because of the high risk of trauma. Rowing, curling, bowling and golfing can also put you in a vulnerable position due to the frequent forward bending that is required.

EXPERIENCED ATHLETE

If you have been playing a sport on a regular basis for a long period of time, you will have developed a certain level of skill and muscle strength to safely perform that activity. Over the years, your bones have developed the strength needed to resist forces placed upon them during this activity. You will be less likely to fracture than a person with the same bone density who did not play this sport.

THE BEGINNER ATHLETE

For older adults, the benefits of regularly playing a sport that you enjoy can far outweigh your risks of falling and fracture. For the beginner, if you have been inactive and want to start exercising or playing a sport, use caution when starting. You must be aware of the risk of high impact movements, the importance of maintaining good posture during the particular activity and know what movements will put you most at risk of fracture.

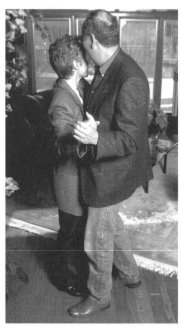

DANCE

Dancing is fun and good exercise. It also has the benefits of being weight-bearing, easy on your joints, good for balance and good for heart and lung fitness. However, when you dance, avoid bending forward, maintain good posture and wear sensible footwear.

WHAT TO DO IF YOU HAVE A FRACTURE

THE SPINE

A spinal fracture is usually accompanied by sudden, severe, sharp back pain. It may be perceived as a muscle spasm. Some describe it as a pulled muscle, while others hear a tearing or popping sound as they lift a heavy object. In many cases a person does not feel pain when the fracture occurs and does not know something is wrong until they wake the following morning.

In 20 percent of all fracture cases, there is no associated pain at the time of the fracture and the person only finds out about the fracture after being X-rayed. If you have a sudden onset of back pain or wake up with back pain, err on the side of caution and see your doctor right away. Or, if you don't have any back pain but have lost height, have a rounded back and have lost the ability to straighten your back, talk to your doctor immediately.

WHAT TO EXPECT IF YOU SUFFER A FRACTURE OF THE SPINE

In the past a spinal fracture meant being confined to a hospital bed for weeks. Today, most people are not admitted to hospital and are cared for at home. Moving in bed, getting in and out of bed and changing positions are usually very painful and the acute (sharp) pain can last for two to twelve weeks.

It is also recommended that during this time, you keep as mobile as possible. If you stop moving for too long a time, your muscles stiffen up and become weaker which will affect your independence. Keeping mobile will also help you minimize loss of strength in your muscles. So get up to go to the bathroom and move around the house. At first, standing up for more than a few minutes or sitting will not be possible. You will also probably need assistance to prepare your meals and to bathe for at least the first week. You will probably need help with more

For older adults, the benefits of regularly playing a sport that you enjoy can far outweigh the risks of falling and fracture.

WHAT TO EXPECT IF YOU HAVE A
FRACTURE OF THE SPINE (cont'd)

demanding activities such as laundry, housework and getting groceries. It's also time to call on your family and your friends. Finally, during this time, you will need to see your doctor regularly for anywhere from a few weeks to as many as twelve weeks, so be sure to arrange for someone to accompany you for these appointments.

HELPFUL AIDS & SERVICES

For the first week or two a rollator walker with four wheels, a raised toilet seat with arms on it and a bath seat can make life a lot easier. Depending on where your bathroom is located, you may also want to have a commode (portable toilet chair) in your bedroom. If your bedroom is not on the same level as the kitchen you may want to set up a bed on the main floor. Beds, walkers and other equipment are available for rental at medical supply companies. There are also many health professionals and resources available to help you and they include the following:

Seek assistance to choose the safest walking aid.

Family Doctor: Pain medication, home care referral, referral to an Osteoporosis Clinic

Physiotherapist: Pain control, selecting walking aids, education and exercises to reduce muscle spasms and stabilize the spine

Occupational Therapist: Assistance with activities of daily living (safest way to perform activities under the circumstances) and equipment: walker, bath seat, raised toilet seat, electric bed, commode and dressing aids

Nurse: Pain control, education, co-ordination of other required resources

Home Support Worker: Meal preparation, bathing/dressing, changing beds, laundry, housework

Other Services: Groceries, meals and prescription delivery services

If you have a stooped forward (kyphotic) posture or a spinal fracture, positioning of pillows can help with comfort.

HIP FRACTURES

The most common cause of a hip fracture is falling. And surprisingly, the hip sometimes fractures first, and the fracture then leads to a fall. Hip fractures are usually accompanied by sudden, severe pain and require an emergency department visit. Fractures are confirmed by X-ray and the person is normally admitted to hospital. Surgery, if required, would be done within the first 24 to 48 hours. Movement is encouraged as soon as possible during recovery and people are encouraged to walk using a walker on the first or second day following surgery. Length of hospital stay varies, and people are usually sent home to recuperate with help from home care services. At the time of discharge, staff at the hospital also provide you with a list of exercises and recommendations on how much you can

HIP FRACTURES (cont'd)

initially move about. The home care physiotherapist will also progress your exercises and help you get back to your previous levels of activity.

It is also important to remember that if you have broken your hip, it is almost guaranteed that you have osteoporosis. After you recover from the fracture, you need to follow up with your doctor about learning strategies to improve your bone mass. Your doctor may order a Bone Mineral Density Test to monitor your bone mass. You should also make sure you are getting enough calcium and Vitamin D as studies in nursing homes have shown that hip fractures drop by 50 per cent when residents receive calcium and Vitamin D supplements.

WRIST FRACTURES

A wrist fracture, also known as a Colles' fracture, usually results from a person falling on an outstretched arm they were using to slow or prevent their fall. Wrist fractures are most common in women aged 50 to 70. The usual treatment for this fracture is casting for six weeks. After the cast is removed, both wrist strength and range of motion are greatly reduced. Daily strengthening and range of motion exercises are necessary to improve mobility and function. Ice and active movement can also help reduce the swelling after the cast is removed.

RIB FRACTURES

Rib fractures are also fairly common. During such fractures, deep breathing, coughing, bowel movements, changing position and moving in bed are all painful. Rib fractures are usually treated conservatively with pain medication, lots of rest and modifying activities. Rib fractures usually take six weeks to heal with the acute pain lasting anywhere from two to six weeks.

Studies show that hip fractures drop by 50 percent when nursing home residents receive calcium and Vitamin D supplements.

PAIN MANAGEMENT

In addition to pain medication prescribed by your doctor, there are several methods to relieve acute pain. A physiotherapist can help you determine what might work best for you. Below is a brief description of some possibilities:

POSITIONING

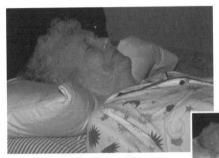

Using pillows under your knees, shoulders, head and arms when lying on your back can relieve stress on the spine and reduce muscle spasm. When lying on your side, a pillow or rolled towel

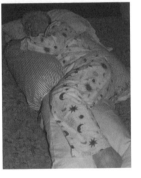

under your waist will prevent the spine from curving and causing pain. A pillow between your knees and ankles will prevent twisting of the spine and improve comfort, while pillows in front and behind you provide support and allow relaxation.

ACTIVITY MODIFICATION

Short-term bed rest, use of appropriate aids such as a walker or bath seat, strategies to conserve energy and getting the appropriate help at home will allow you the time you need to heal.

ICE

A soft ice pack or ice massage (stroking the area of pain with ice) works as a local nerve block and provides temporary relief during the acute pain stage. Ice can be applied to the points of burning and numbness every hour.

HEAT

After the first two to seven days, heat can provide soothing pain relief, especially if there is muscle spasm. Moist heat is best but microwavable hot packs and heating pads also work well. Be careful not to burn yourself by lying too long on an electric heating pad. Hot packs that will gradually cool off (especially if you are likely to fall asleep) are much safer to use.

MASSAGE & MYOFASCIAL RELEASE

Gentle massage or myofascial release (technique performed by a physiotherapist or registered massage therapist) can relieve pain and muscle spasm.

ULTRASOUND

Therapeutic use of sound waves can help relieve pain, reduce localized swelling and promote healing. Ultrasound machines (see adjacent picture) are portable and can be used in your home by your home care physiotherapist if necessary.

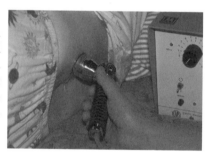

TENS

Transcutaneous Electrical Nerve Stimulation (TENS) is a battery-powered electrical unit that transmits small electrical signals through electrodes placed on the skin where the pain is located. The electrical signals block the pain. Usually pain relief lasts as long as the machine is worn, however, the effect can last much longer by reducing muscle spasm. A physiotherapist can advise you on appropriate use.

EXERCISE

Deep breathing exercises promote relaxation and isometric exercises (tightening of muscles without movement) can help reduce muscle spasm and support the back. Mobility and range of motion exercises help keep you mobile and reduce stiffness.

IN SUMMARY

Although osteoporosis is often referred to as the silent thief, we now know that there are simple steps we can take to keep this thief in check.

Keep your diet rich in calcium with adequate Vitamin D. There is an abundance of natural sources of calcium available to us through a variety of beverages and food. If you think you are not meeting your daily requirement, consult your doctor or dietitian; calcium supplements may be necessary.

Exercise is the recurring theme behind prevention of many key diseases, such as heart disease, stroke, diabetes and osteoporosis. By remaining active, including weight-bearing exercises, we build and maintain stronger and better bones.

Menopausal women are faced with a unique situation where their rate of bone loss substantially increases in association with their lack of estrogen. This puts them at greater risk than men for osteoporosis and fractures. Be sure to consult your doctor and learn about your special needs.

And remember, good posture, whether you are sitting, standing or moving protects your body from muscle imbalances, injuries and pain. Sit upright, stand upright and, when lifting, tighten your abdominal muscles and bend at your hips and knees keeping your back straight.

Get down to the basics, build better bones and enjoy the quality of life you deserve - now and in the future.

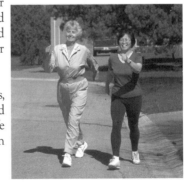

BIBLIOGRAPHY

BOOKS

1. Health Canada, Nutrient Value of Some Common Foods, Canadian Government Publishing, 1999.
2. Hilborn, Kathy, Driver's Back Manual: An Ergonomic Guide to Injury Prevention, Injury Reduction Systems, A Division of Alberta Back School Inc., 1997.
3. Lazowski, Darien-Alexis, Boning Up On Osteoporosis for Physiotherapists, Course Manual, 1999.
4. McKenzie, Robin, Treat Your Own Back, Spinal Publications Ltd., New Zealand, 1985.
5. Nelson, Miriam, Ph.D., Strong Women, Strong Bones, Putnam and Grosset, 2000.
6. Roberts, Scott, Fitness Walking, Indianapolis, Masters Press, 1995.
7. Sahrmann S., Diagnosis/treatment of muscle imbalances associated with regional pain syndromes, Course Manual, 1990.
8. J.P. Bilezikian, J. Glowacki, and C.J. Rosen, eds., The Aging Skeleton, Academic Press, 1999.

JOURNALS

1. Chow, R., Harrison, J., Relationship of kyphosis to physical fitness and bone mass on post-menopausal women, American Journal of Physical Medicine Rehabilitation, 66, 219-227, 1987.
2. Dietary Reference Intakes for Calcium, Phosphorus, Magnesium, Vitamin D, and Fluoride, Pre-publication, The National Academy of Sciences and Institute of Medicine, National Academy Press, 1997.
3. Gregg, E.W., Cauley, J.A., Seeley, D.G., Ensrud, K.E., Bauer, D.C., Physical activity and osteoporotic fracture risk in older women, Study of Osteoporotic Fractures Research Group. Ann Intern Med, 129:81-88, 1998.
4. Gower, Timothy, HEALTH, Is Calcium The Key to Strong Bones?, March 2000.
5. Helmes, E., Hodsman, A.B., Lazowski, D.A., Bhardwaj, A., Crilly, R., Nichol, P., Drost, D., Vanderburgh L., Peterson, L., A questionnaire to evaluate disability in osteoporotic patients with vertebral compression fractures, Journal of Gerontology: Medical Sciences 50A(2):M91-M98, 1995.
6. Hanley, David, Josse, Robert, Prevention and Management of Osteoporosis: Consensus Statements From the Scientific Advisory Board of the Osteoporosis Society of Canada, Can Med Assoc J 155-(7), Oct., 1996.
7. Itoi, E., Sinaki, M., Effect of back strengthening exercise on posture in healthy women 49 to 65 years of age, Mayo Clin Proc Nov., 69(11):1054-9,1994.

8. Jam, Bahram, The Jam Report, The Diaphram Muscle … Vital for life and stability, Vol. 1, Number 4, January 2000.

9. Lactose Intolerance or Milk Allergy? Nutrition Communications, Dairy Farmers of Ontario, 1998.

10. Lazowski, D.A., Hodsman, A.B., Helmes, E., Howe, D., Carscadden, J., Thoracic kyphosis and back extensor strength in elderly osteoporotic women, Proceedings of the 24th Annual Scientific and Educational Meeting of the Canadian Association on Gerontology, 101, October 26-29, Vancouver, B.C., 1995.

11. Osteoporosis Society of Canada, Osteoporosis Update, Vol.3 No.4. Fall 1999.

12. Sinaki, M., Itoi, E., Rogers, J., Bergstralh, E., Wahner, H., Correlation of back extensor strength with thoracic kyphosis and lumbar lordosis in estrogen deficient women, Am J Phys Med Rehab., Sept/Oct., 75(5):370-4 1996.

13. Sinaki, M., Effect of physical activity on bone mass, Curr Opin Rheumatol. Jul. 8(4):376-83, 1996.

14. Sinaki, M., Mikkelsen, B., Postmenopausal spinal osteoporosis: flexion versus extension exercises, Arch Phys Med Rehab., Oct. 65(10):593-6, 1984.

15. Waters, T., Anderson, V., Garg, A., Fine, L., Revised NIOSH equation for the design and evaluation of manual lifting tasks, ERGONOMICS, Vol. 36, No. 7, 749-776, 1993.

16. Osteoporosis Society of Canada, Clinical practice guidelines for the diagnosis and management of osteoporosis, Can Med Assoc J, 55:1113-1129, 1996.

HELPFUL RESOURCES

1. North American Menopause Society
http://menopause.org/consedu/index.html

2. Osteoporosis Society of Canada
http://www.osteoporosis.ca/corporate/c04.html
(1-800) 463-6842 or (1-416) 696-2817

3. National Osteoporosis Foundation
http://www.nof.org/prevention/prevention.htm
(1-800) 223-9994 or (1-202) 223-2226

4. National Institute of Health, Osteoporosis and Related Bone Diseases (National Resource Center)
http://www.osteo.org/health.html
(1-800) 624-BONE

5. International Osteoporosis Foundation
http://www.osteofound.org/what/index.html

THE PERFECT GIFT THAT SHOWS YOU CARE!

BODY BASICS *for bones*, Beat osteoporosis, build better bones! makes a great gift for all generations because it's never too early nor too late to protect you and your family. A book filled with evidence-based and practical information for everyone. Build better bones and enjoy the quality of life you and your loved ones deserve. It's great for Christmas, for birthdays, graduations, Mother's Day, Father's Day or any day of the year! Check your local bookstore or order directly from us.

TO COMPLEMENT BODY BASICS *for bones*...

Simple and healthy products, as featured in this and other BODY BASICS books, are available through Birchcliff Publishing Inc. These convenient and inexpensive products are designed to relieve and prevent pain.

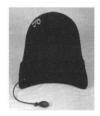

BACK SUPPORT:
EmbraceAirPlus fully adjustable back support. Vertically adjustable bladder for a personalized fit. Easy squeeze bulb to adjust firmness. Attaches to existing seating - ideal for your home, office and car.

BACK PILLOW:
LumbAirPlus fully adjustable back pillow. Easy squeeze bulb to adjust firmness. Lightweight and portable - ideal for your home, office or travel.

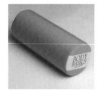

LOWER BACK ROLL:
Cylinder-shaped foam supports your natural inward curve and improves your posture. Lightweight and portable - ideal for your home, office and car.